Essential Oils

30 Essential Oil Skincare & Beauty Recipes

Table of content

Introduction

Beauty and skin care products should be as natural as your body. Why put a factory-made cosmetic or product on your skin? It contains mysterious chemicals not even listed on the label. Have you ever wondered where those chemicals go, after the lotion or cosmetic has "worn off"? Well, the pores in your skin absorb them. Your body and skin then reads those chemicals as foreign matter! How many cells will be damaged in the process of eliminating that nasty stuff from your body? It takes the skin and body a long time to rid itself of that which does not belong inside of you.

In this book, there are recipes for making your own essential oils. That is far better because you can control the quality and strength of the oils you make. It is also a much cheaper way of doing it, and will save you money. You can even grow your own crop of herbs and beautiful flowers for use in the moisturizers here and usage in their pure form. Of course, these crops will enhance the beauty of your yard.

The fragrance of these essential oils is mesmerizing. It has a calming effect in its own right. What's more, the recipes in the following chapters were designed to be simple and inexpensive.

Moisturizers are vital in keeping your skin supple and soft to the touch. The recipes in this book will provide you with superb skin care. In addition, the anti-aging properties of many of these natural beauty mixtures are recommended for all, and should be used around the edges of the eye (where "crow's feet" form), on your "smile wrinkles", and on your neck. As you grow older, the tendons of the neck begin to protrude, unless your skin is kept moist and soft. The time to start treating for that occurrence is when you are young.

The Citrus Essential Oils

Health benefits of citrus oils have been known and used for centuries. They have strong antibacterial and antioxidant qualities. Essential oils also aid in keeping your skin blemish-free. Practitioners of ancient Ayurvedic medicine believed in maintaining a healthy balance of body fluids, and skin purification facilitates that process. Skin can be rejuvenated by the astringent properties of the citrus essential oils. Cleansing the pores in your skin permits it to "breathe" and expel the toxic substances within your body caused by bodily process and the environment.

The Essential Oils from Flowers

Oils derived from flowers have a tranquillizing effect on your spirits, and disinfect the skin and face simultaneously. Naturally, it is pleasant to smell the sweet perfume as you move through your hectic day. Lavender essential oil is superb as a skin-cleansing agent. Patchouli has been used since ancient times for treating dry skin, acne, and dandruff (when used on the scalp). Rose essential oil is considered an antidepressant. After all, when you smell a rose, it immediately relaxes you! Rose oil has also been correlated with prevention of viral and bacterial infections. Geranium oil is wonderful for oily skin and its psychological benefits include the reduction of anxiety. It also makes your skin look radiant. The procedures for making essential oils not only apply to the flowers in this book, but also to other flowers, fruits, and herbs.

The Herbal Essential Oils

As an example of the health benefits of organic herbal oils, sweet basil is known to alleviate fatigue and has distinct digestive properties. It reduces muscle cramps and even earaches! Thyme essential oil will tone your skin, prevent acne and facial blemishes, and it has anti-aging properties. Chamomile has long been known as an organic tranquilizer. The herbal essential oil recipes here can be adapted to other herbs you grow in your particular region.

Chapter 1 – Make Some of Your Own Essential Oils for Recipes

The recipes in this book can be made using your own homemade essential oils, or you may buy them online or at a health store. Sometimes they are sold at booths at craft shows. This particular Chapter presents recipes for a few essential oils you can make at home. The methods for making these essential oils can be used to make other essential oils you may like to try. The process is the same for all of them.

1. LEMON ESSENTIAL OIL

Lemon essential oil may be used for the recipes below, or as an astringent in its pure form. *Beware!* Lemon Oil and Grapefruit Oil (next recipe) tend to increase the photosensitivity of your skin. It is not recommended that you expose yourself to too much sun following use. If your skin is particularly sensitive, you should use the recipe for orange essential oil instead.

Ingredients: ¼ - ½ cup olive oil or safflower oil

1 lemon

cheesecloth

Instructions:

Peel the lemon. Grate the white underside of the peel. Place the lemon peel and olive oil in an 8 oz. jar. Place a folded piece of cheesecloth over the top and cover. Shake the jar vigorously.

Put the jar into a pan of water. Boil the water. Lower the heat and simmer for 2 hours. Store it in a dark pantry closet, shaking the mixture often. It is recommended that you store it for 3-6 weeks for a strong solution.

In its pure form, it is a very strong astringent, and a cleanser for your skin. Lemon oil mixes well with other essential oils. It is used with some of the skin care recipes in this book.

2. GRAPEFRUIT ESSSENTIAL OIL

Ingredients: ½ cup olive oil or safflower oil

1 grapefruit

cheesecloth

Instructions:

Grate the grapefruit peel. You might want to cut off the white underside of the grapefruit peel rather than grate it. This is especially applicable if you are using a "winter" grapefruit, which has a much thicker underside. Otherwise, the grating process will take too long. Put the peel into a jar with the olive or safflower oil and shake it vigorously. Take the cheesecloth and put a folded piece of it over the jar. Close the jar. Store in a cool dark place for 5 weeks.

Like the lemon essential oil, grapefruit essential oil in its pure form is an astringent. The grapefruit has terrific detoxifying properties for your skin.

3. ORANGE ESSENTIAL OIL

This oil is to be used in some of the beauty and moisturizer products you are going to make, following the recipes listed here. It may also be used in its pure form for those who are more sensitive to sunlight and would rather not use the lemon or grapefruit essential oil. It is a mild astringent when used straight from the jar. It is also an antibacterial agent, and has the property of improving circulation. You can substitute it for other essential oils, or combine it with them, if you wish. Orange essential oil is very compatible with other homemade organic beauty products.

Ingredients: ½ cup safflower oil

1 orange

cheesecloth

Instructions:

Peel the orange. Save some of the pulp. Grate the orange peel as best you can. Press the orange pulp to extract some juice. Put the orange peels, juice and safflower oil in a jar with a lid. Place the jar in boiling water. Turn it down to simmer. Let the mixture simmer for 3 minutes. Pour it into a jar with a lid. Put a folded-up piece of cheesecloth between the jar and the lid. Close the lid. Shake. Let sit for 3 days and shake it up occasionally.

4. THYME ESSENTIAL OIL

Thyme essential oil can be used in pure form to help rid yourself of blackheads. It is also useful for skin scars. Herbs, utilized as ingredients, make remarkable skin care products.

Ingredients: ¾ cup thyme leaves

1-cup olive oil

Instructions:

Use a ceramic container that has a cover. Do not use metal. Stuff the leaves in it. Pour enough olive oil in it to cover all the leaves. Be sure that no leaves are floating on the top. Cover the mixture. Let it stand for 3 days. Shake the container often to aid in the release of the essential oils from the thyme. Store in a dark, cool place. Many recommend a 3-week period before you first use it. After that time has elapsed, separate the oil from the leaves using a colander. Pour the oil-thyme solution into a glass container. That is your essential oil. Use it with your recipes. Thyme essential oil is very versatile.

5. SWEET BASIL ESSENTIAL OIL

Sweet basil essential oil is used as a cleansing product for the face, neck and skin. It may be used in its pure form, as here, or added to one of the other recipes, such as those for moisturizers.

Ingredients: ¾ cup sweet basil leaves

1-cup olive oil

Instructions:

Use a ceramic jar or container to make your essential oil. Put the leaves into the olive oil. Be sure no leaves are floating on top of the olive oil. Cover it. Shake it up and store in a dark place. Your food pantry is fine. Check it frequently and shake it up. After 2-3 weeks, it should be ready. Test it out. Pour out a very small amount of the olive oil-basil mixture and smell it. If it doesn't have a strong leafy fragrance, store it longer. Strain the mixture to separate the leaves from the oil mixture, and place the solution in a small jar to use in your recipes.

6. PATCHOULI ESSENTIAL OIL

Patchouli essential oil can be used in pure form for spreading on dry or chapped skin. It is sweetly aromatic.

Ingredients: ¾ cup patchouli flowers

                1-cup safflower oil

Instructions:

Place the flowers in a jar with a lid. Fill with the safflower oil and tighten lid. Shake it a number of times. Let stand for 7 days in the sun, shaking vigorously and often. Strain the mix to separate the flower heads from the oil. Reserve the leftover flowers and oil. If the scent is not pervasive enough, repeat the procedure until the fragrance strengthens. For patchouli, it may require a longer period of time to pull the essential oils out of the flower heads. Once you are satisfied with the scent, separate the flowers from the safflower oil-patchouli solution. Pour into small jar. You may use this as your essential oil in the recipes.

Store the unused patchouli petals in your refrigerator for other uses, such as in your baths.

7. CHAMOMILE ESSENTIAL OIL

Chamomile essential oil, used in its pure form, makes an ideal skin cleanser and wrinkle remover. It helps with acne, skin rashes, and rosacea. Chamomile essential oil can even be used to lighten blonde hair! Mix it with the shampoo recipes in this book, or add it to your regular shampoo.

Ingredients: 1 cup chamomile flowers

¾ cup olive oil

1-tablespoon vitamin E

½ tablespoon rosemary essential oil

Instructions:

Put the flower heads in a jar. (You might have extra flowers that you can save for use at another time) Cover the flower heads with olive oil. Put a lid on it and shake vigorously. Place the jar in a pot of boiling water. Turn off the heat and permit the essential oil in the chamomile flowers to extract into the olive oil. Remove from the stove. Add the rosemary oil and vitamin E. Permit it to reach room temperature. You might want to use it right away in the recipes, or you can store it in a sunny location for later. That will increase its strength.

Note: Chamomile essential oil may be used on a poultice for your eyes at night. It has anti-aging properties, and will decrease the number of wrinkles that form on your eyelids and below your eye. Always test an eye product first to determine if there will be any allergic reaction.

8. ROSE GERANIUM ESSENTIAL OIL

Rose Geranium essential oil can be used in pure form to smooth your wrinkles and promote the elasticity of your skin. This is also a good anti-aging product and perfect for skin care.

Ingredients: ¾ cup rose geranium flowers

1-cup safflower oil

5 drops lavender essential oil

Instructions:

Prepare as you would chamomile essential oil. (above) Use it in the recipes. It may also be added as a fragrant oil to mix with other essential oils.

9. LAVENDER ESSENTIAL OIL

Lavender essential oil is excellent as an anti-aging product. It is needed for some of the recipes here, but can also be added to other recipes, as you wish. It smells beautiful and can be used in your house on the carpets.

Ingredients: ¾ cup lavender flowers

1 cup sunflower oil

Instructions:

Place the flowers in a jar with a lid. Fill with the sunflower oil and tighten the lid. Shake it a number of times. Let it stand for 5 days in the sun, shaking the mix vigorously and often. Strain the mixture, reserving the flowers and oil. The scent should be pervasive, but – if not, repeat the process. Store in a sunny location.

10. ROSE ESSENTIAL OIL

Rose essential oil is wonderful for dry and aging skin.

Ingredients: 1½ cups rose petals

½ cup sunflower oil

3 drops rosemary essential oil

2 drops vitamin E

Instructions:

Put the petals in a jar. Reserve the extra petals. Cover the petals with the sunflower oil. Put lid on it and shake. Place the jar in a pot of boiling water. Turn off the heat and permit the essential oil to extract into your oil. Remove. Add the rosemary oil and vitamin E. Permit it to reach room temperature. You might want to use it right away, or you can store it in a sunny location for use in the recipes. It can enhance the essential oils when used in combination with other essential oils.

ROSE PEAR POTPOURRI

Take the extra rose petals from your recipe above. Add to a pot of boiling water. Peel and cut up half a pear. Place it into pot and let the water continue to boil. Add more water if needed. Lower the temperature to simmer, and you will have a wonderful fragrance permeating your home. Great for guests!

Chapter 2 –Recipes for Facial Masks, Eye Masks, and Moisturizing Lotions

FACIAL MASKS –

First, A Word about Honey

Honey is famous for its antibacterial properties. It is an organic product, of course, and used by honeybees to protect themselves and their young from infection. Although some recommend raw honey, even the refined version of honey is fine for use in facial masks.

11. HONEY FACE MASK

Ingredients: 1 tablespoon raw honey

3 drops of lavender essential oil

Instructions:

Combine ingredients. (Doesn't it look luscious?) Dampen your face and apply. It may seem rather wet. If so, just dab it with a hand towel.

12. AVOCADO FACE MASK

Ingredients: 1/3 cup grated cucumber (no peel)

1 avocado, mashed

¼ teaspoon lemon essential oil

Instructions:

Combine all of the ingredients in a bowl. Refrigerate it for 30 minutes. Remove and let the mixture reach room temperature. Apply to your face, a little bit at a time. Then build it up, until you reach the desired amount.

EYE MASKS –

These recipes are specifically intended to reduce or remove wrinkles around the eyes.

Note: When you use any homemade product around or on the eyes for the first time, always test it out first for any signs of redness. The eyes and the skin areas around them are very sensitive.

13. HONEY-POTATO EYE MASK

Ingredients: ½ potato, grated

2+ teaspoons honey

Instructions:

Mix both together to make a paste. You might want to use your blender if necessary. Apply around your eyes at night.

14. GRAPEFRUIT-APPLE EYE MASK

Ingredients: 1/8 cup grapefruit juice

1/8 cup apple juice

2+ teaspoons honey

Instructions:

Mix all together and apply around the eyes.

Note: *Test for sensitivity to the citrus acid in the grapefruit first.*

15. COTTAGE CHEESE EYE MASK

Ingredients: 1/8 cup cottage cheese (small curds)

2 drops coconut oil

2 drops almond oil

2+ teaspoons honey

Instructions:

Mix very well in your blender until the cottage cheese is smooth. (curds not visible). Add the coconut oil, almond oil, and honey. Apply around the eyes.

MOISTURIZERS –

..... A Word about Shea Butter, Coconut Oil, and Almond Oil

Shea butter is a major ingredient of many of the moisturizer recipes listed below. Cleopatra used it! According to the archeologists, shea butter was carried in caravans into ancient Egypt where it was prized for its usefulness for skin care and it has healing properties as well. Shea butter is totally organic, having been extracted from the nuts of the African shea tree. Therefore, shea butter is a botanical fat, not an animal fat. The Egyptians also used it as a protection against the harsh sun and dry hot winds that blew in from the Sahara desert to the west of the country. Medicinally, it is used as a base for ointments and has anti-inflammatory properties.

Coconut oil is noted for its use in skin care. It is an effective moisturizer, prevents dryness and flakiness, and noted for its anti-aging properties.

Almond oil contains such healthful components as potassium, vitamin E, zinc, and proteins. All of those organic properties make it ideal for use for skin care. Once absorbed through the skin and circulated throughout your body, it has health benefits for your heart as well.

Note: *Keep all moisturizers refrigerated when not in use. You may bring your moisturizers to room temperature before applying if you wish.*

16. COCONUT LOTION

Ingredients: 1 tablespoons coconut oil

½ cup shea butter

5 drops rose geranium essential oil

5 drops of lavender essential oil

Instructions:

Melt the shea butter. Add the coconut oil and stir. Remove from the heat. Pour it into a bowl and put it into your freezer to cool. (about 15 minutes) Do not allow it to harden, so be sure to check it occasionally. Add rosemary and lavender oil and whip it all together. Apply the lotion to your face and neck areas...your hands too, if you like.

17. MYRRH VANILLA LOTION

This recipe is great for dry or chapped skin. It also has antioxidant properties that are antibacterial and it has been known to decrease skin cancer risk.

Ingredients: 1 tablespoons myrrh essential oil (or one of your own)

¼ cup sunflower oil

½ cup shea butter

5 drops vanilla extract

Instructions:

Melt the butter. Leave some lumps in the butter. Add the myrrh oil and vanilla extract. Stir. Place it into your electric mixer bowl and beat it for a short time. Some bits of butter may still show. That is good. Turn the mixer on high to incorporate more air into it. Put it into your jars and cover tightly. Let it stand a few days until the mix hardens slightly. It is ready to use.

18. FRANKINCENSE LOTION

This beauty recipe is recommended for aging skin. It also aids in reducing wrinkles and "crow's feet".

Ingredients: 2 teaspoons frankincense essential oil

                ¼ cup coconut oil

                1-cup shea butter

Instructions:

Melt the butter. Add the coconut oil and stir. Remove from heat and add the frankincense. Pour it into a bowl. Cover. Cool in the freezer, but do let it freeze. Remove it and let it cool down to room temperature. It is ready to apply.

19. SANDALWOOD LOTION

This recipe is recommended for dry skin. It has an aromatic and woody scent.

Ingredients: 3 teaspoons sandalwood essential oil

¼   cup olive oil

1-cup shea butter

Instructions:

Melt the butter only slightly. Beat by hand or in electric mixer. Do not overbeat. Add the olive oil *slowly* and add the sandalwood oil. Stir by hand until it is the right consistency for use.

20. NEROLI ORANGE LOTION

This is excellent for getting rid of stretch marks, and also for aging skin.

Ingredients: 1 teaspoon neroli essential oil (or one of your own)

2 teaspoons orange essential oil (use your recipe above)

¼   cup coconut oil

¾ cup shea butter

Instructions:

Melt the butter only slightly. Add the coconut oil and stir. Add the neroli essential oil and the orange essential oil. Stir by hand until it is the right consistency for use.

21. LAVENDER LOTION

This is excellent for getting rid of stretch marks, and also for aging skin.

Ingredients: 3 teaspoons lavender essential oil

¼   cup coconut oil

¼   cup shea butter

Instructions:

Heat the shea butter and coconut oil over low heat until some shea butter still has particles in it. Remove from heat. Add the lavender essential oil. Place it you're your freezer for a little while, checking on it frequently. When the mixture has nearly solidified, remove and let it return to room temperature. As it reaches room temperature, watch the consistency. When the right texture and consistency is reached, you may use it.

22. LILAC LOTION

This is an all-around lotion for moisturizing any skin type.

Ingredients: 5 drops lilac essential oil (or one you made yourself)

1-teaspoon vitamin E

¼ cup aloe vera juice or aloe vera water (optional)

1 cup grated beeswax*

¼ cup almond oil

¼ cup water

Instructions:

In a bowl, place the aloe vera juice, vitamin E, and the lilac essential oil. Stir and set aside. Mix the grated beeswax and oil. It will be lumpy. Put the beeswax and oil in a glass jar and set it into a pot of water. Boil the water, and then reduce it to its lowest setting. When the beeswax is entirely melted, remove it from the stove. Beat all of the ingredients in an electric mixer at the lowest setting. Put it into the freezer to cool, checking on it frequently. When the mixture is cool, remove it and bring it back to room temperature. You may apply it now. The remaining lotion should be stored in the refrigerator.

*Obtain beeswax from a local beekeeper. It is also sold at craft shows at the honey booth, or on the Internet.

23. JASMINE CLEANSING LOTION

This lotion is effective for dry skin. It is especially useful in the winter when your house is very dry.

Ingredients: 1/8 cup olive oil

1-tablespoon shea butter

1-teaspoon vitamin E oil

½ cup shaved glycerin soap

¼ cup almond oil

¼ cup water

2 drops jasmine essential oil (rose essential oil may also be used)

Instructions:

Place a jar or glass-measuring cup in a pot. Place the soap, butter, and olive oil in the cup. Heat until the soap, butter, and oil melt. This may take a little while. Put it into a blender and add the water, vitamin E, and jasmine essential oil. Blend at slow speed. The water may separate from the rest of the mixture. If this happens, repeat the process until both are thoroughly blended. Put it on high speed if necessary. Pour it out of your blender and let it stand for 24 hours. The mix will thicken in time. Be patient!

24. ROSE LOTION

This is an all-around moisturizing lotion. It has a hypnotic fragrance.

Ingredients: ¾ cup shea butter

¼ cup almond oil

4 drops rose essential oil

Instructions:

Mix shea butter and almond oil as best you can. Place it in a glass jar or measuring cup. Put it into a pot of water. Boil. Reduce the heat and let it cool. Add the rose essential oil. Put it into your freezer. Remove it before it is completed hardened. Put it into an electric mixing bowl and whip it at high speed. Spoon out the product when it is fluffy and put the mixture into a jar. Keep it stored in the refrigerator when not in use.

Chapter 3 – Body Scrubs, Shampoos, and Eye Shadows

25. HONEY-ORANGE BODY SCRUB

Ingredients: 2/3 cup soft soap of your own choosing

                  ¼ cup honey

                  2 teaspoons almond oil

                  1-teaspoon vitamin E

                  2 teaspoons liquid vegetable glycerin

                  6 drops orange essential oil (recipe is in Chapter 1)

Instructions:

Gently blend all the ingredients. This is a simple one!

26. SUGAR LEMON BODY SCRUB

Ingredients: ½ cup brown sugar

                     ½ cup coconut oil

                     5 drops lemon essential oil

                     2 drops vitamin E

Instructions:

Mix all ingredients. Rub the mix on your body and rinse. This will exfoliate your skin. It smells sweet and delicious!

27. SANDLEWOOD SHAMPOO

This is magnificent for oily hair!

Ingredients: 1 cup water

¼ cup cornstarch

¼ cup rubbing alcohol

5 drops sandalwood essential oil (or chamomile essential oil as in Chapter 1)

Instructions:

Mix all of the ingredients together. Be sure the cornstarch is totally blended into the mixture. Wash your hair as usual.

28. SWEET BASIL SHAMPOO

Sweet basil is well known as a cleansing agent. This will boost the effectiveness of the other ingredients. This can be used in conjunction with the flower essential oils in the other recipes if you wish.

Ingredients: ¼ cup almond oil

¼ cup liquid Castille soap

4 drops sweet basil essential oil (as in Chapter 1)

Instructions:

Combine all of the ingredients in a bottle and vigorously shake. Wash you hair as usual.

29. COCOA EYE SHADOW*

Ingredients: cocoa powder (for brown shades) or activated charcoal (for darker shades)

dab of shea butter and a drop of coconut oil

Instructions:

Mix together small amounts of the ingredients until the color and texture meet your expectations. Apply.

Test out any homemade eye shadow first. Do this by putting just a tiny dab on your eyelid. Give it some time to see if you have any reaction. The eyes are a very sensitive area. Be sure all the ingredients are very clean.

30. NUTMEG EYE SHADOW

Ingredients: ground nutmeg (for lighter reddish-brown shades)

        1-2 drops of coconut oil

        ½ teaspoon cornstarch

Instructions:

In a small Pyrex dish, put in the cornstarch. Add the oil slowly. Stir in the ground nutmeg with a toothpick until you have the desired color. Apply.

Chapter 4 – The Importance of Skin Care in Overall Health

Your skin is the largest organ in your body and allows for interaction between your body and the environment. Every pore in your skin absorbs air, but our air is not pure air composed of oxygen, nitrogen and other inert elements. Pollen, pollution, airborne gases, methane, sawdust, soot, ozone, dust, excessive sunlight, water vapor, and microscopic particles emitted from decaying matter infiltrate the air you are exposed to. Daily you are assaulted with that! Protection of your skin is vital, or these substances will enter your body through your skin.

If you look at the skin of an infant and compare it with your own, the difference is visibly noticeable. Your skin loses its suppleness with age, and becomes prone to developing blemishes, bumps, and wrinkles. This is especially true of your face, which has the greatest exposure. Sometimes people's faces form blackheads, acne, rashes, dryness and discoloration. You don't see that on baby's faces. All of the environmental exposure you experience throughout your life has long-reaching effects on your overall health. That is why skin care is so important. The usage of organic essential oils and ingredients will assure you that no additional foreign matter or pollutants enter your body through the skin.

Cleansing

Everyone needs to wash their body daily, but they need to wash their faces and hands even more often. Those areas are unprotected by clothing. You cleanse yourself to wash away the noxious bacterial substances that cling to your body and face. As cleaning agents, organically based compounds are far superior to the chemical products manufactured for skin care. Those factory-made products contain the very pollutants you are trying to wash off!

Nature has its own organic way of cleansing. Have you ever seen a dirty chickadee or blue jay? All animals have the instinct to clean themselves. I once watched a dusty groundhog run through a patch of tall grasses, and run out of the patch dust-free. He used the wet clean grass to clean his fur! You too can take advantage of Mother Nature's beauty pantry. These recipes have presented ingredients from only organic sources without additives or chemicals created in a laboratory.

Pores in your skin become clogged because they undergo a buildup of dirt and foreign matter. Using cleansers derived from essential oils and natural organic sources will do the job effectively and efficiently. Your body will also benefit from the medicinal properties of plants and flowers.

Moisturizing

Exposure to the air results in dryness, as the oils in your body evaporate with the heat and wind. If you have oily skin, your natural bodily oils will absorb unwanted particles that need to be washed first before you apply moisturizers. In the body, essential oils are absorbed very rapidly. If you feel "greasy," that sensation will subside once your skin has absorbed all the ingredients in the organic products. All of the components in the recipes above are healthy for your body, and helpful as they circulate throughout your entire body.

Moisturizers serve the purpose of preserving suppleness and natural beauty to your skin. They can "plump it up" to disguise wrinkles. The astringents, such as those found in the citrus essential oils, will tighten up your skin in areas where there is "sagging". They also soften the skin, so that it is pleasant to the touch. Rough areas on your face and neck will be made smooth due to the oils used in these recipes.

Chapter 5 – The Functions of the Skin

Your skin is more complex than appears at first glance. There are 3 main layers of cells that compose it. The outermost layer, the epidermis, is just the top layer. Many cellular structures lie beneath it and need nourishment, moisturizing, and cleansing. The ingredients, like shea butter and the essential oils recommended here are absorbed into the skin. Those and all the other components have properties that aid in cellular replenishment. Under the epidermis, there are capillaries, nerves, sweat glands and oil glands, hair follicles, membranes, and even muscles. The recipes above will provide you with the substances that nourish each of the layers of the skin. By-products of those ingredients are carried via the capillaries to other areas of the body. No one wants foreign matter and manufactured chemicals to be transported throughout the body. That only causes harm and damage.

Using these organic skin care and natural beauty treatments will produce a wholesome you. There are solutions in these recipes for dry skin, oily skin, blemishes, and wrinkles. Essential oils complement and support structures in the skin such as the glands in the dermis (under the epidermis) of the skin. The moisturizers in the recipes fortify the capillaries and membranes of the cells there. Many of the recipes contain ingredients that are antioxidants, and provide your body with a tool to liberate your body from free radicals, a cancer-causing molecule. The cleansing nature of the recipes will alleviate stress and uplift your spirits. After using them for a while, you will see a change in your skin. It will be more supple, more glowing, and more beautiful.

Conclusion

These recipes gave you a foundation to explore the wondrous effects of using organic ingredients for your skin including essential oils, and organic products only. You have treated yourself to Mother Nature's way of handling your body's needs for rejuvenation. You have discovered that the pampering of natural products and organic solutions is the best way to combat the assault by an environment of impure substances and unwanted toxins. Essential oils delight your skin and perform magical effects on your emotions. They smell as fragrant as a field of flowers and herbs. Harsh manufactured substances only introduce minerals and factory-made chemicals that irritate the skin. You have discovered that organic beauty solutions can and do work. No doubt, after you have tried just a few recipes, you have wondered why we haven't been using them all along.

www.ingramcontent.com/pod-product-compliance
Lightning Source LLC
Chambersburg PA
CBHW071154280526
45787CB00003B/1502